Happy Buys

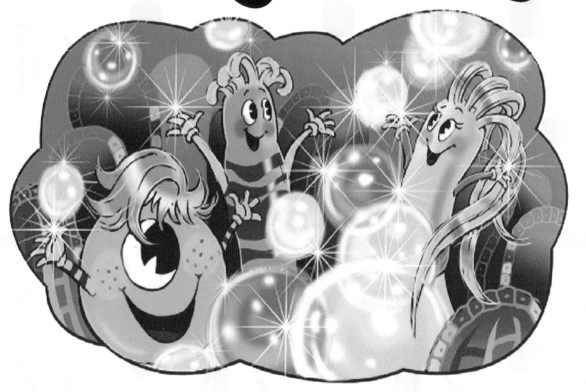

by Erin Hankinson and Scott Hankinson MD
Illustrations by Eva Vagreti

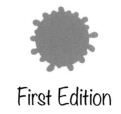
 happybugsbook and Bugman_md

 ™HappyBugsBugs and @HappyBugs2022

www.Happy-bugs.com

The book you are about to read may have the most valuable information for your family on the topic of nutrition.

Over the past 15 years, medical science's knowledge regarding the importance of the Microbiome and Whole Food Plant Based eating (WFPB) has exploded. As the technology of genetic sequencing has developed, so has the understanding of how important the "bugs" in our body are. Collectively this is referred to as the microbiota and how it influences our genes, the microbiome. It is estimated that over 90% of our genes can be influenced by what we put in our mouth. The study of this is referred to as Epigenetics

As a physician, this is quite different from what I was taught and believed for decades. The fact that we can influence the outcome of our gene expression with diet, is revolutionary.

As my personal knowledge of the microbiome has developed, I've come to regret the way my own children were raised with regards to diet. With this in mind, my wife and I decided to write a fun book to educate children (as well as their parents and grandparents) about their own "bugs", and how the food choices they make influence the way those bugs function and affect our health.

My prayer is that you will find this a fun and delightful book that will stimulate you and inspire you to educate yourself about your "happy bugs". Along those lines, you can reach out via email or social media for references and further information.

Erin and Scott Hankinson MD

November, 2022

Words to Look for

ENDOTOXIN
A molecule present inside bacterial cells that are released with cell death. They are very inflammatory. LPS is an example of an endotoxin.

FIBER
A type of carbohydrate that the body cannot digest. It is broken down by our "bugs" to produce small chain fatty acids.

MACROBIOTA
A term referring to the bacteria, yeast and viruses that live on and inside of our bodies.

MACROMIOME
A term for the collective gene pool made up of the microbiota.

MUCIN LAYER
A protective layer on the bowel. It is part of the "gut barrier".

PREBIOTICS
A term for the "food" consumed by the microbiota, such as fiber and resistant starch, that cannot be digested in the small intestine.

PROTEIN
A structure made up of amino acids that is used to make structures in the human body.

SMALL CHAIN FATTY ACID
Metabolites produced by the microbiota or "bugs" in the large intestine. These are made through the fermentation of dietary fiber and resistant starch. The three most common are: Acetate, Butyrate and Propionate. All three are very anti-inflammatory and are used for many cellular functions including cell energy and mucin production. They also cross the blood brain barrier and are thought to be essential to mental health.

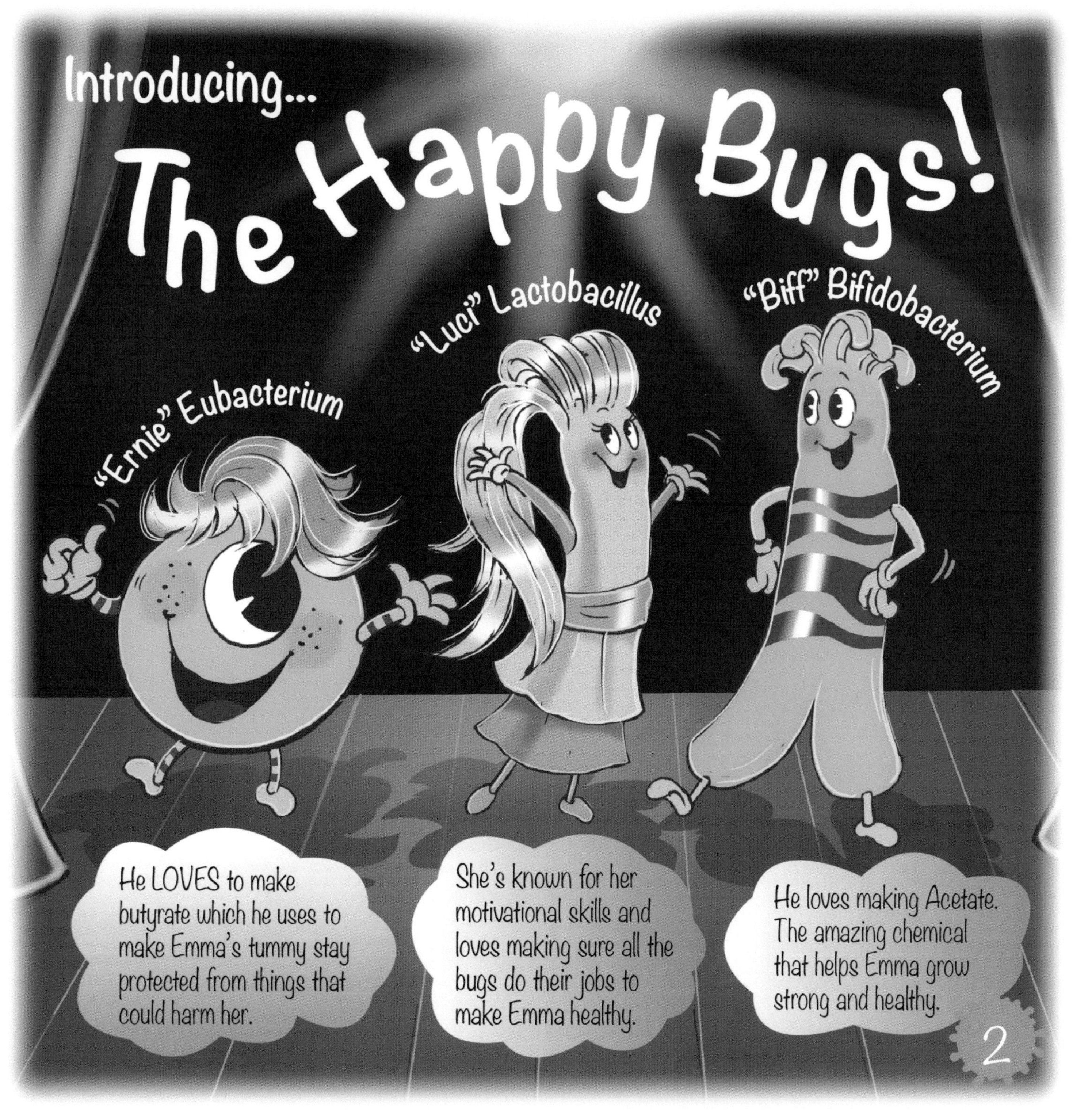
Introducing...
The Happy Bugs!
"Ernie" Eubacterium
"Luci" Lactobacillus
"Biff" Bifidobacterium
He LOVES to make butyrate which he uses to make Emma's tummy stay protected from things that could harm her.
She's known for her motivational skills and loves making sure all the bugs do their jobs to make Emma healthy.
He loves making Acetate. The amazing chemical that helps Emma grow strong and healthy.

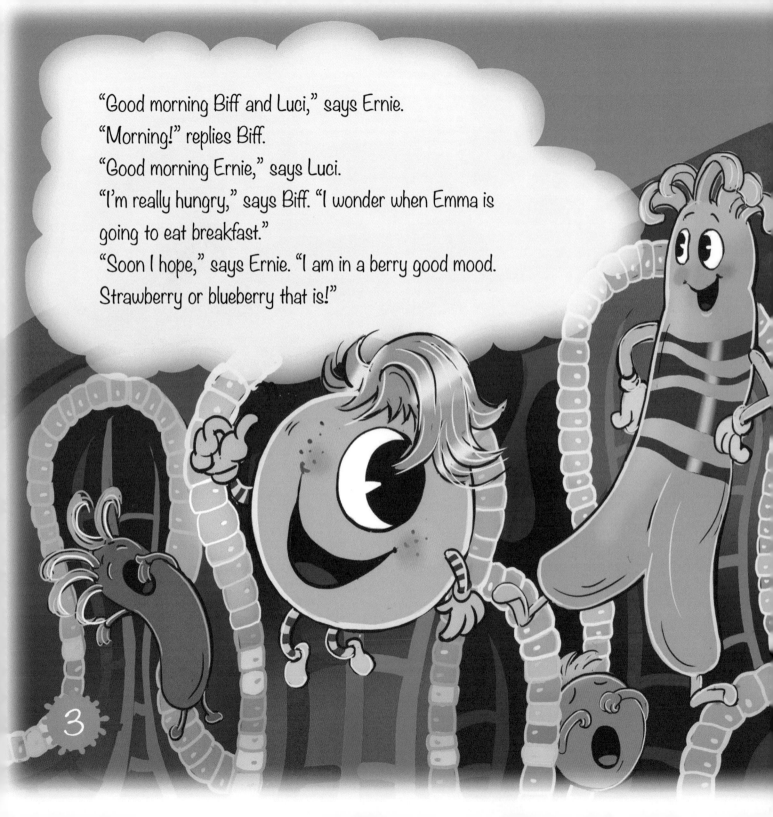

"Good morning Biff and Luci," says Ernie.

"Morning!" replies Biff.

"Good morning Ernie," says Luci.

"I'm really hungry," says Biff. "I wonder when Emma is going to eat breakfast."

"Soon I hope," says Ernie. "I am in a berry good mood. Strawberry or blueberry that is!"

3

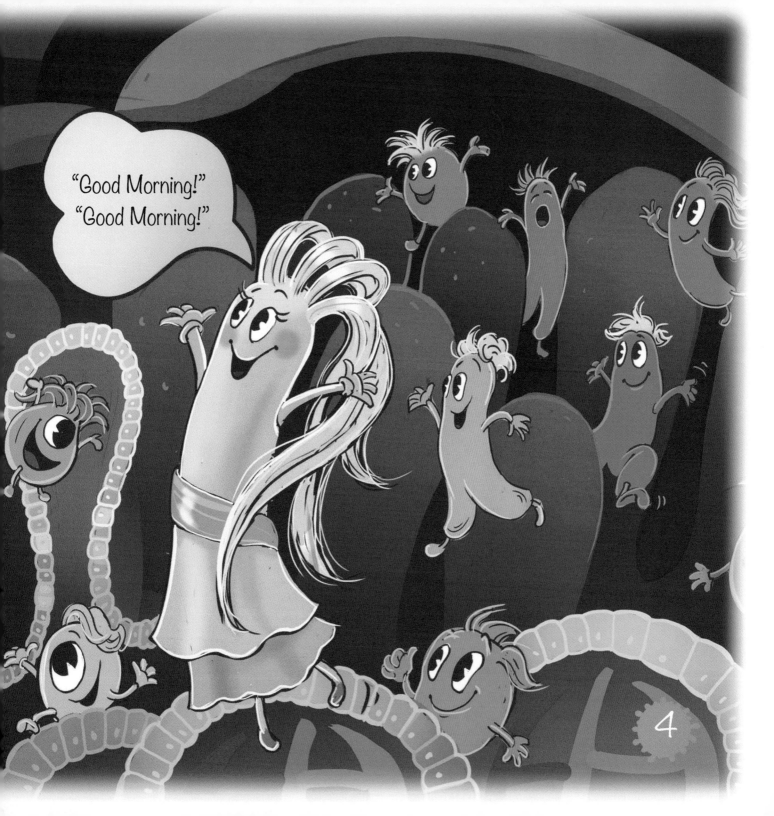

"Good morning sweetie," says Emma's dad.

"I see you are all dressed. Did you brush your teeth?"

"Yes Dad," she answers. "Is my oatmeal almost ready?"

"Just a few more minutes. I need to add some soy milk and chia seeds. How about some strawberries too?" asks Dad.

"Yummy. Yes please," says Emma.

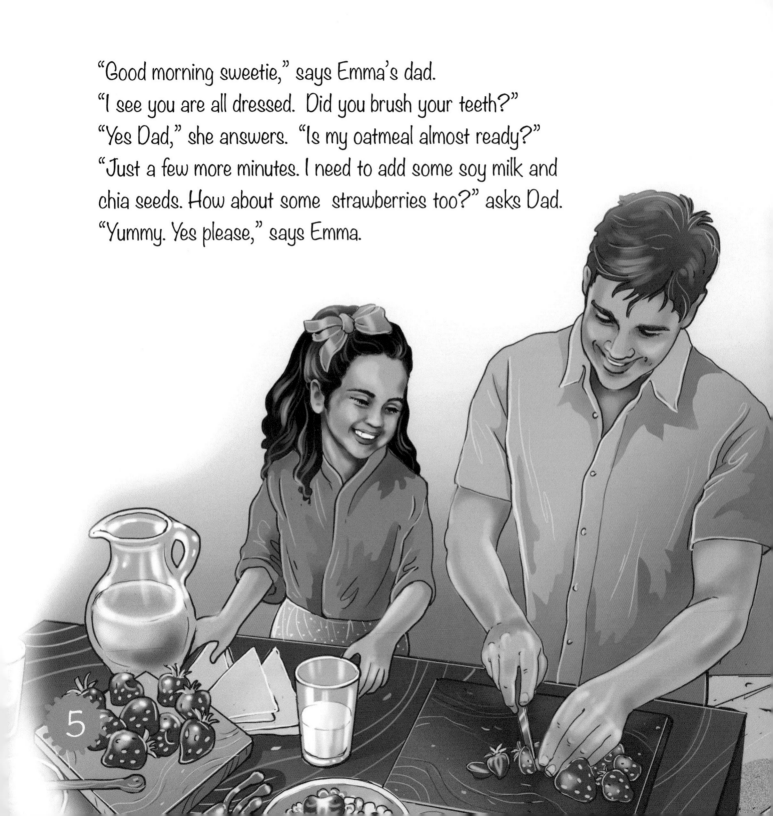

5

Mom enters the kitchen and sees a table nearly ready for breakfast.

"What a beautiful rainbow of colors I see! Thanks for preparing everything. You guys are really making great food choices!"

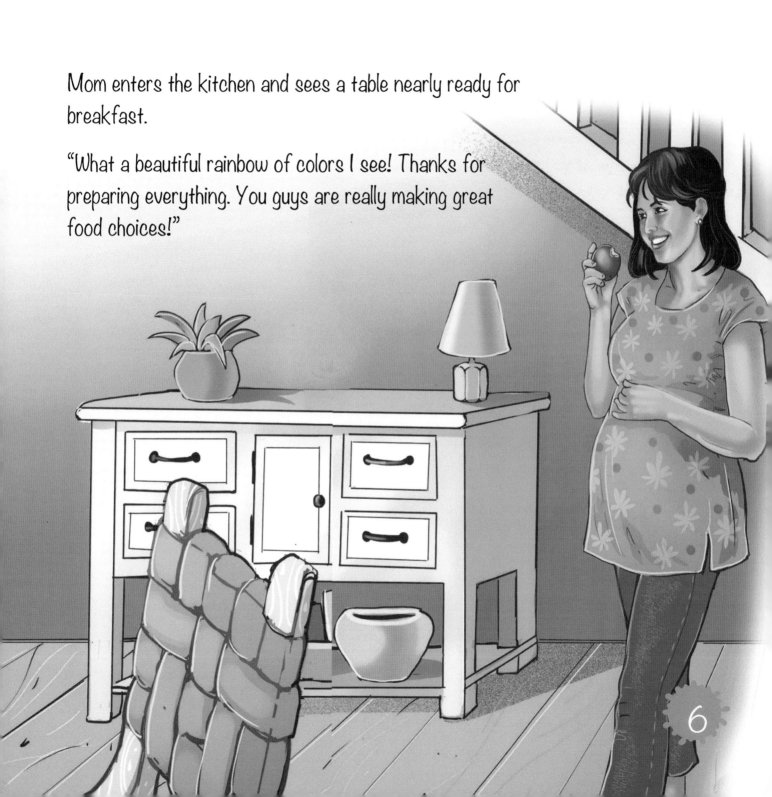

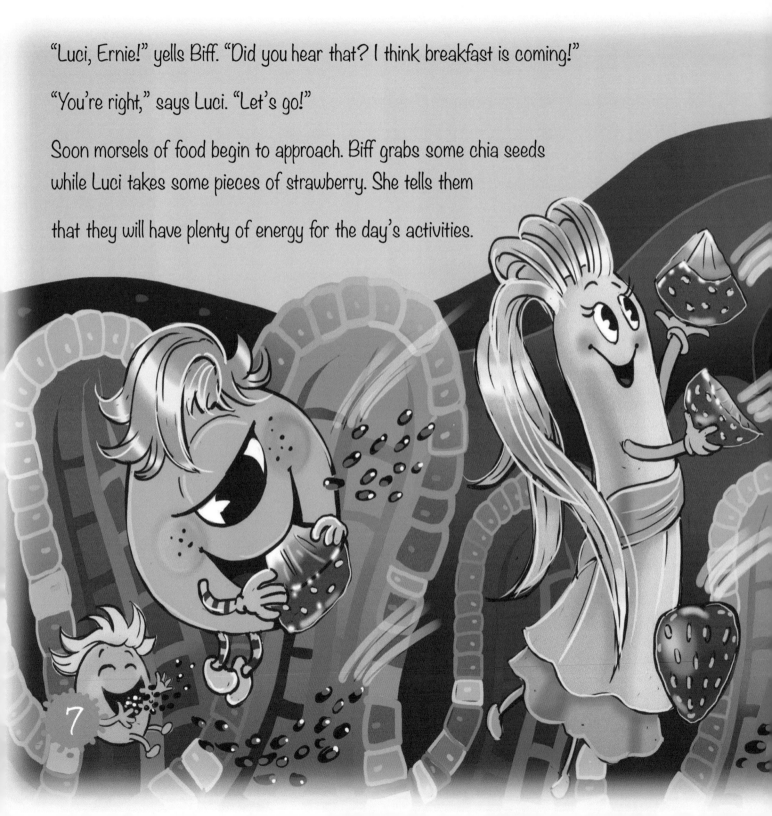

"Luci, Ernie!" yells Biff. "Did you hear that? I think breakfast is coming!"

"You're right," says Luci. "Let's go!"

Soon morsels of food begin to approach. Biff grabs some chia seeds while Luci takes some pieces of strawberry. She tells them

that they will have plenty of energy for the day's activities.

7

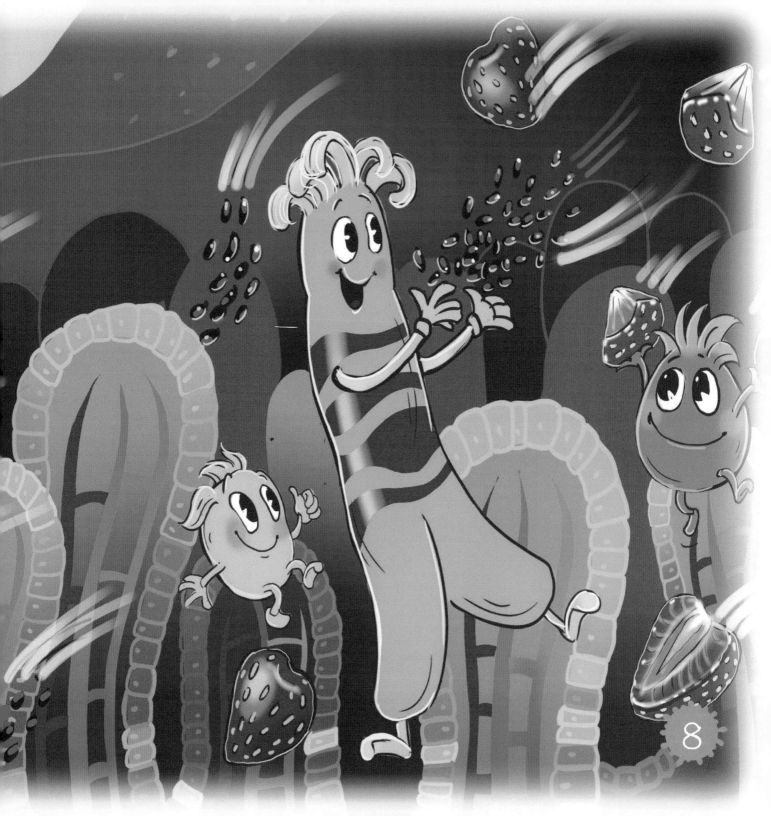

8

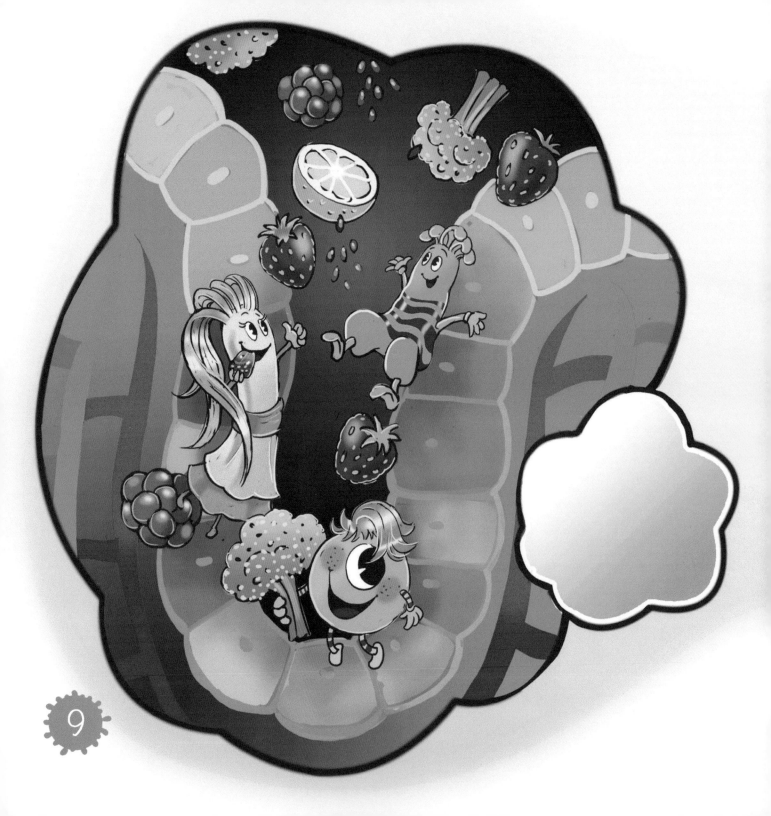

"How is your oatmeal, Emma?" asks Dad.

"Great!" she says. "I love the little chia seeds. They like to stick to my teeth."

"I bet your belly bugs love them too!" says Mom.

"I have bugs in my belly?" asks Emma.

"Yes," explains Mom. "They're very small, but very important. We couldn't live without them."

"Really?" Emma asks.

"Exactly," says her father. "Our bugs eat whatever we eat, kind of like your baby brother growing inside Mom's tummy. Whatever Mom eats, he eats."

"That's right," says Mom. "When we eat the kinds of foods high in fiber, our bugs make their own babies AND have energy to do their jobs."

Emma looks curiously at her dad. "What kind of jobs?"

"Well, when your bugs have enough energy, they make things your body needs to help you grow up strong and stay healthy."

Mom joins in and points out that our good bugs do not like to eat junk food.

"If we get full on sugary snacks and greasy foods our good bugs go hungry and we feel yucky."

11

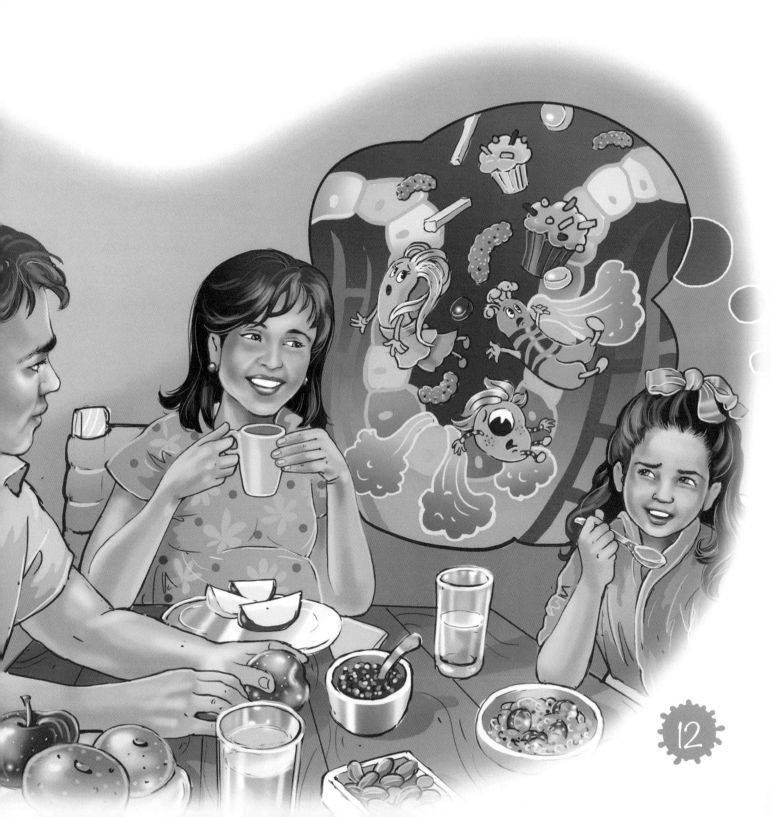

12

Luci stands up tall and announces,
"It's time to get busy! I'm making **PROPIONATE**.
Biff, can you focus on ACETATE?"

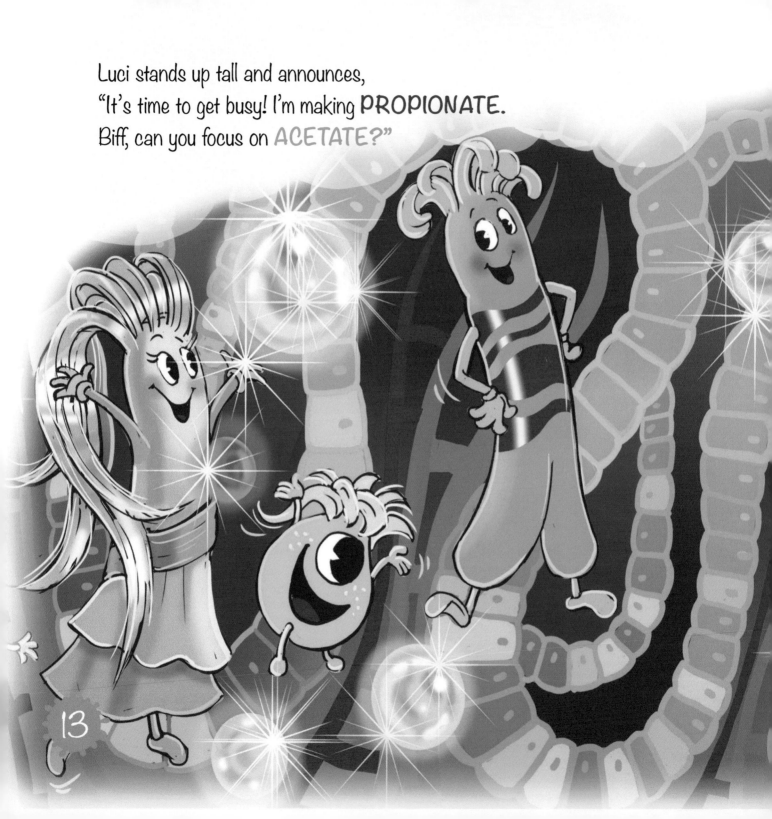

13

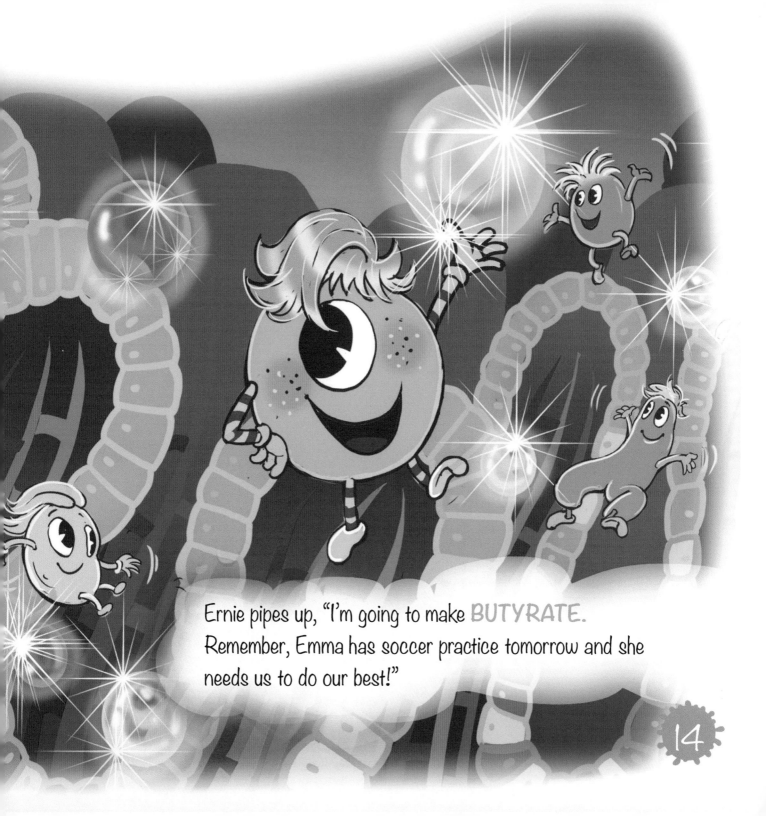

Ernie pipes up, "I'm going to make BUTYRATE. Remember, Emma has soccer practice tomorrow and she needs us to do our best!"

14

"Wow, Emma! You were really fast out there on the soccer field," says Coach.
"Thanks!" says Emma.

"It's because my bugs are strong and doing a good job."

"Your bugs? What bugs?"

"My belly bugs," Emma replies.

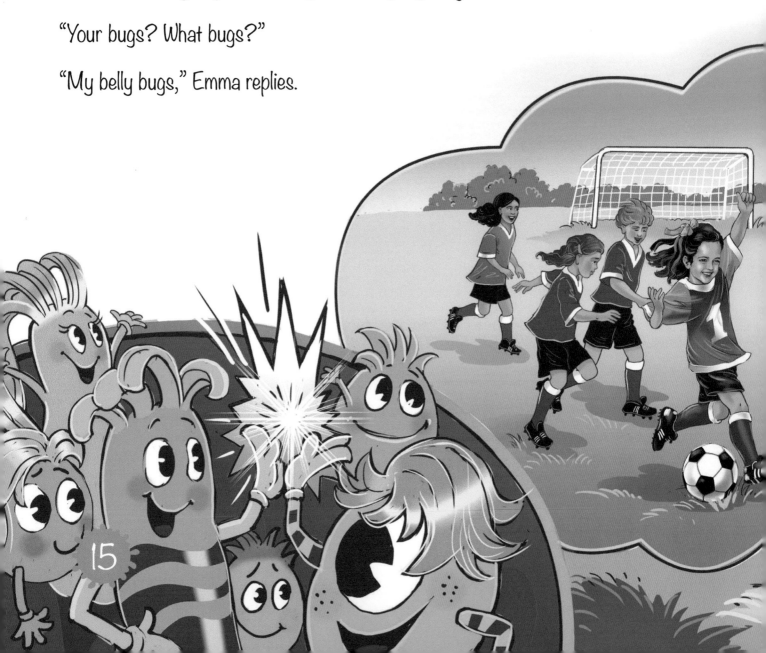

"Did you eat bugs for breakfast?" Coach asks.

"No, silly. I ate fruit and oatmeal so my belly bugs can make me run really fast and ..."

"Oh, those kinds of bugs," Coach replies. "You really are smart for kindergartner."

Emma smiles up at coach proudly.

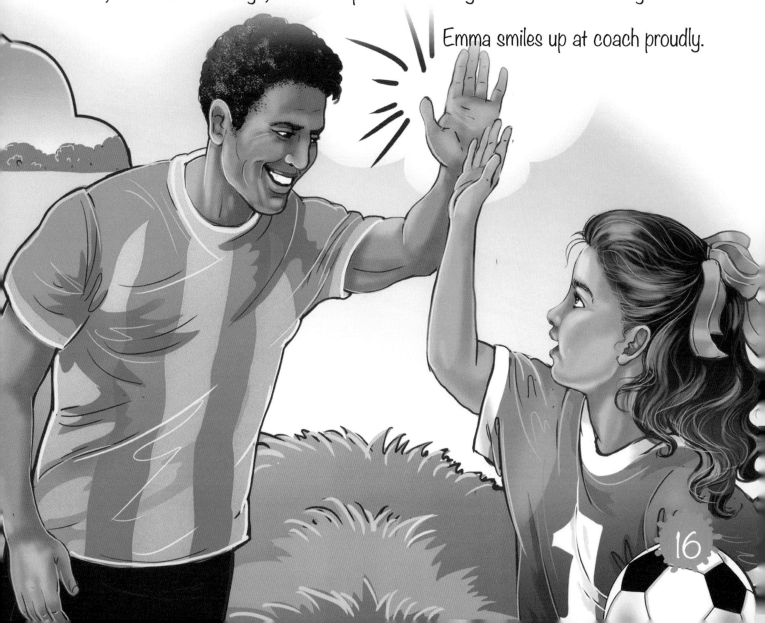

16

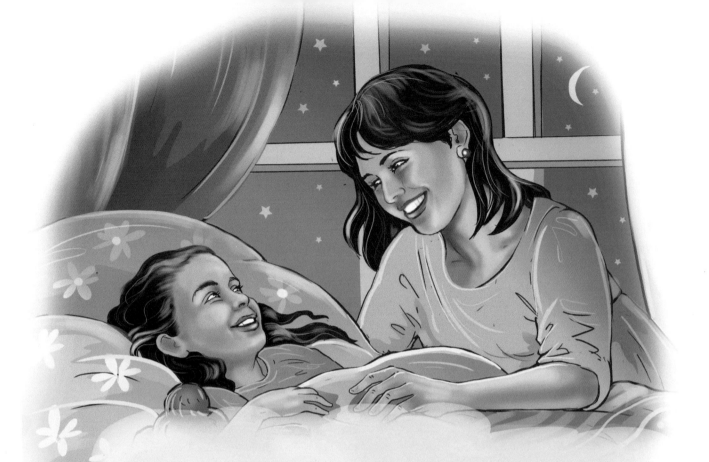

"How was soccer practice?" asks Mom.

"It was great! Coach said I was running fast and doing really well."

"You can thank your belly bugs for that," says Mom. "You need to get some sleep now. Your bugs do better when you get a good night sleep. Remember, tomorrow is your friend Luke's birthday party."

17

"Luke's party is going to be so much fun! He's having a bouncy house with a slide and everything!" says Emma.

"Wow!" says Mom. "That sounds like fun! I am glad you and Luke have become good friends. He is a very nice boy."

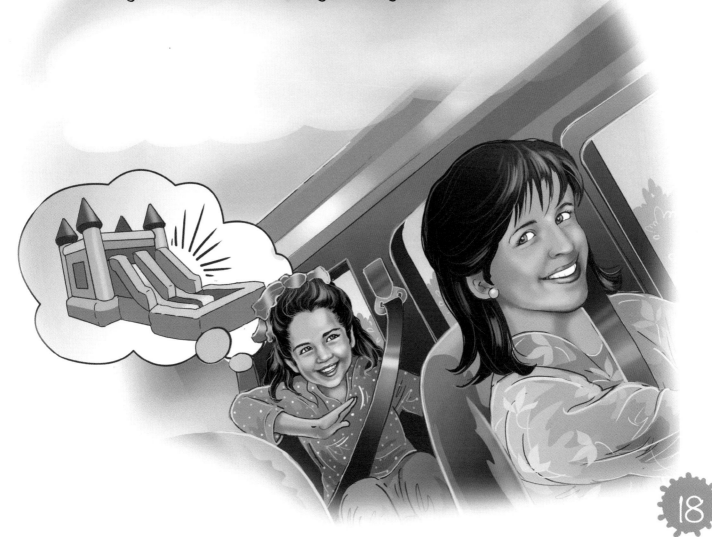

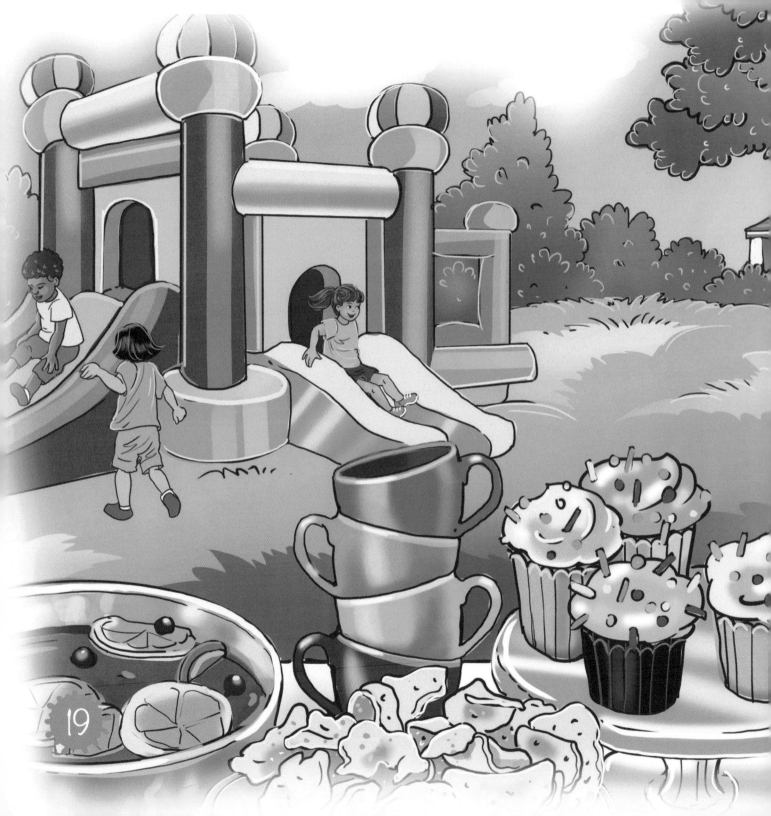

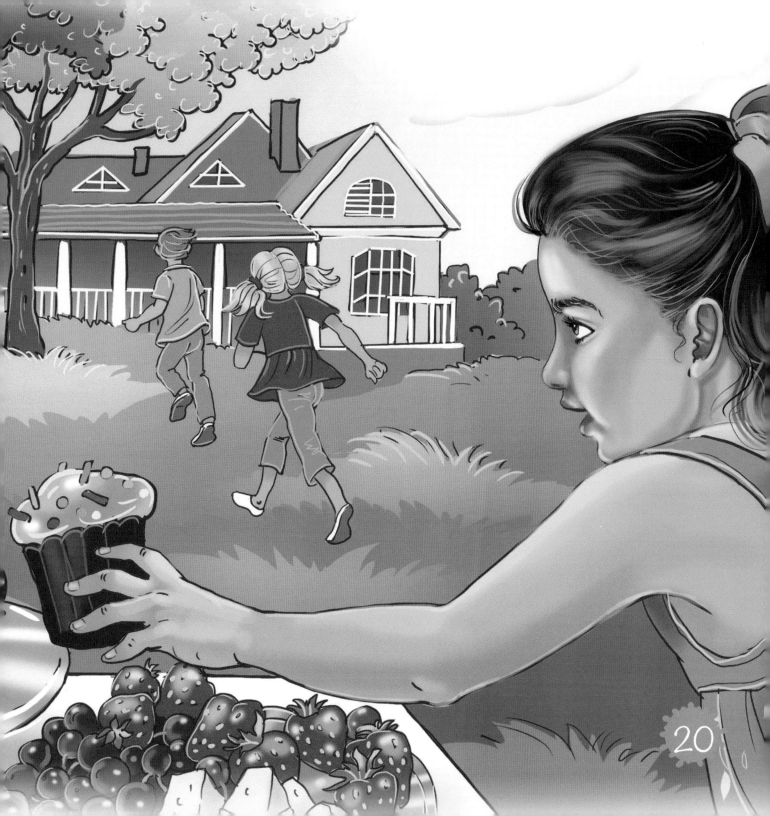
20

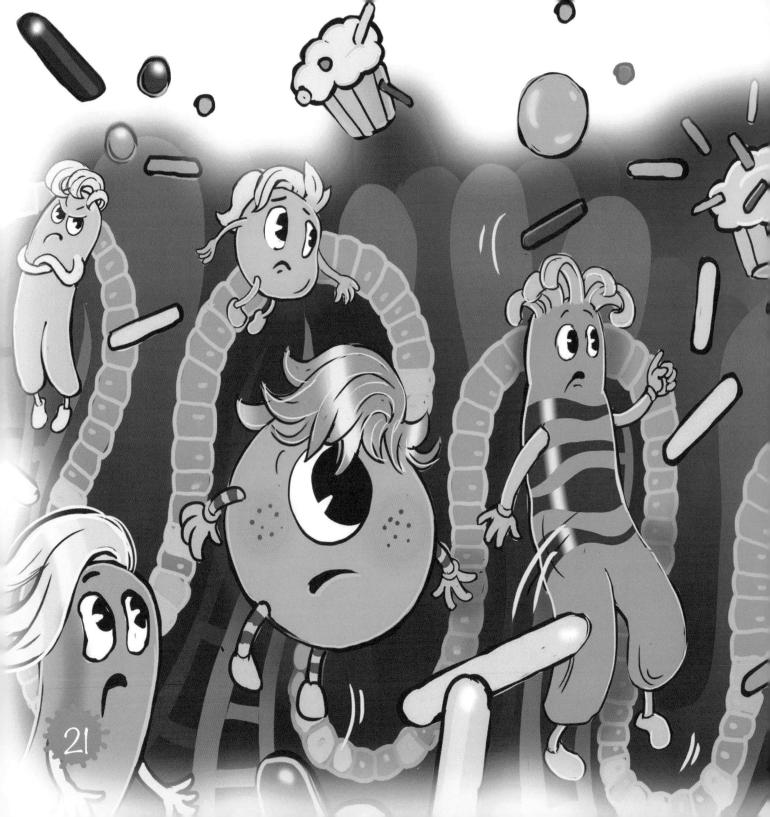

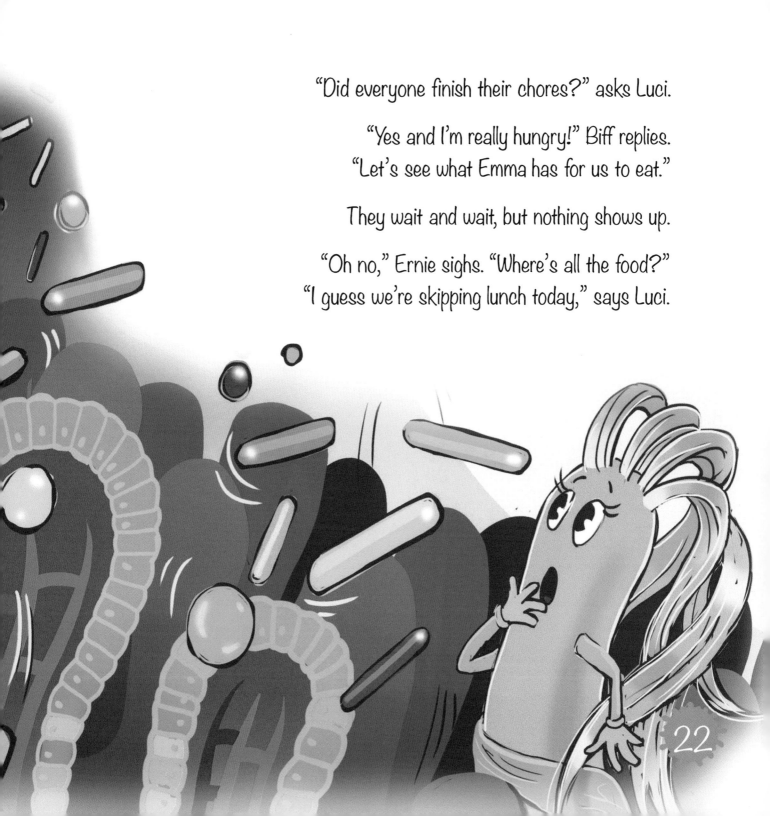

"Did everyone finish their chores?" asks Luci.

"Yes and I'm really hungry!" Biff replies.
"Let's see what Emma has for us to eat."

They wait and wait, but nothing shows up.

"Oh no," Ernie sighs. "Where's all the food?"
"I guess we're skipping lunch today," says Luci.

22

Emma's dad yells from the kitchen. "Remember, in a few hours we're riding bikes to the park for a cookout with the Hendersons!"

"Aw Dad, I do not feel like it," says Emma.

"But you love biking," says her dad. "That's not like you. Are you feeling all right?"

Before Emma could answer her mom spoke up. "Luke's Mom told me Emma only ate cupcakes at the party. She didn't even touch the tray of fruit I brought."

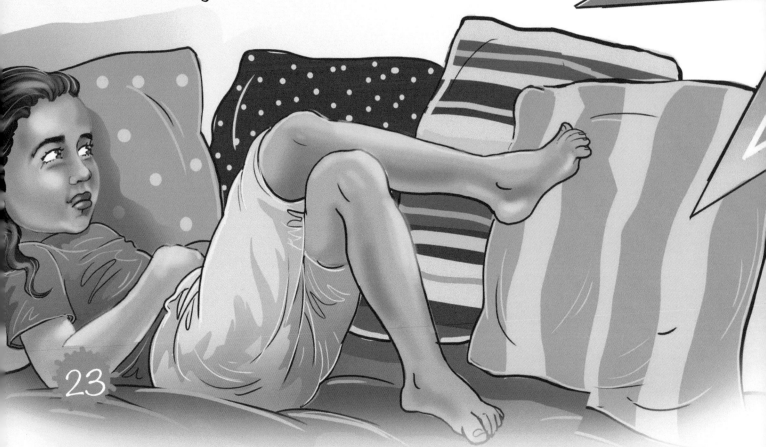

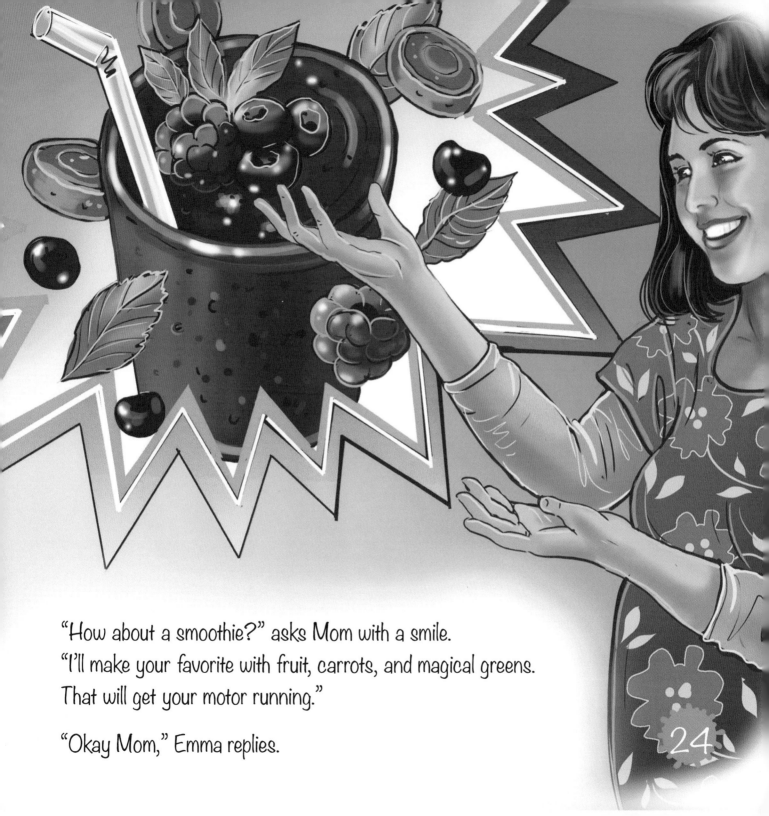

"How about a smoothie?" asks Mom with a smile.
"I'll make your favorite with fruit, carrots, and magical greens.
That will get your motor running."

"Okay Mom," Emma replies.

24

"Wow Emma!" says her dad. "Look at you! That smoothie really did the trick!"

"I know, Dad. My bugs and I are working hard and I'm not even tired. They really are my friends."

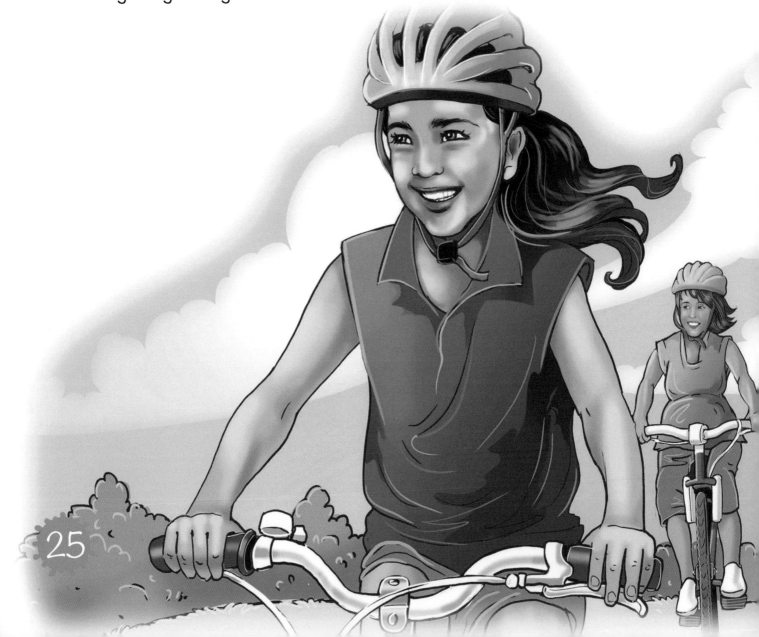

25

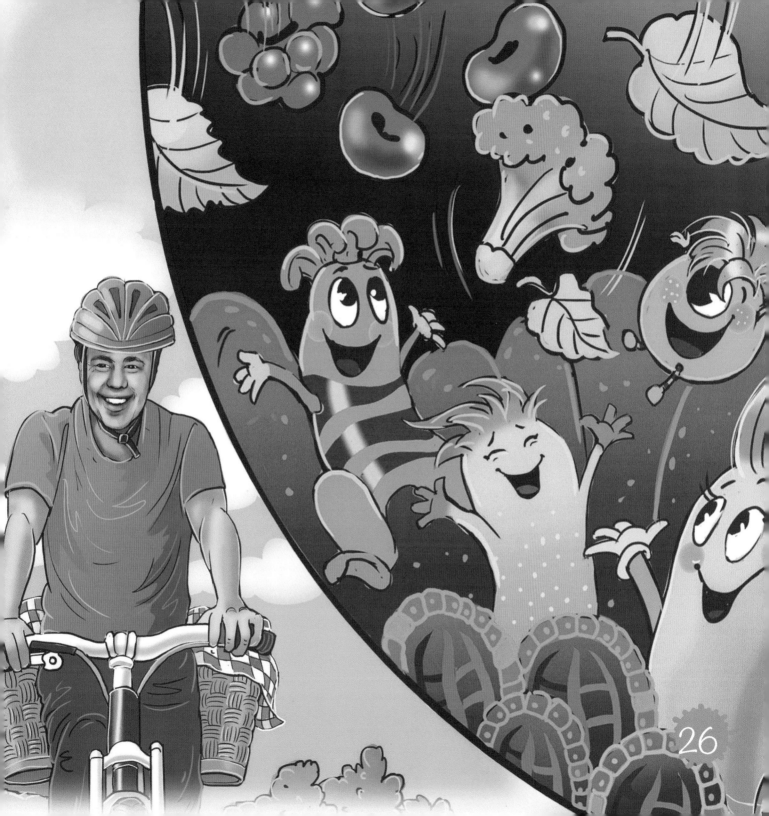

26

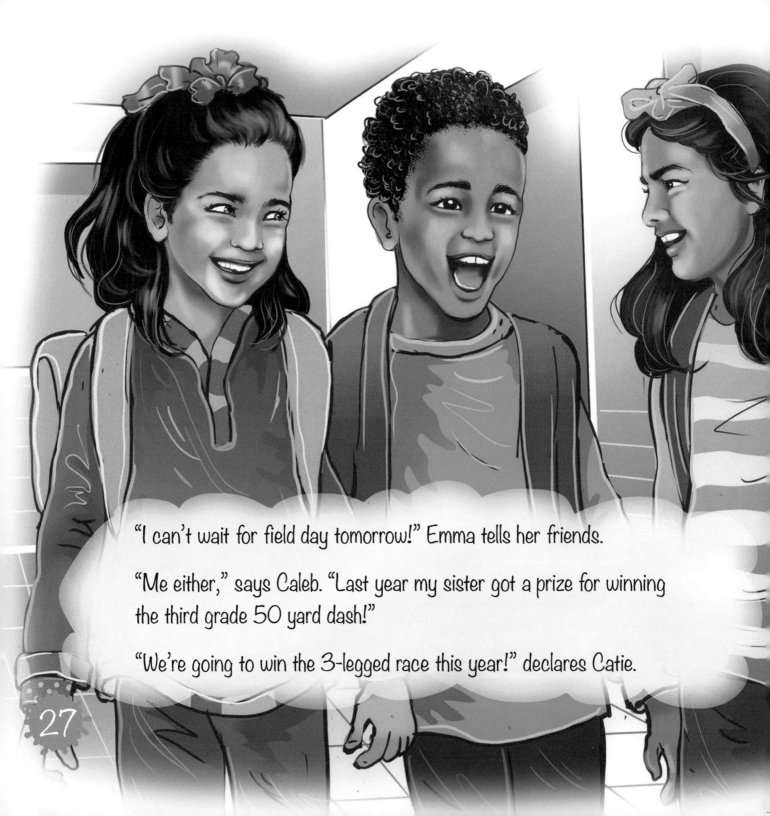

"I can't wait for field day tomorrow!" Emma tells her friends.

"Me either," says Caleb. "Last year my sister got a prize for winning the third grade 50 yard dash!"

"We're going to win the 3-legged race this year!" declares Catie.

The following day Emma and her mom are in line at the concession stand during field day.

"Mom," says Emma, "I really want some cotton candy. Do you think my bugs would like it?"

"I don't think so honey. If you want to win the 3-legged race your bugs will need healthy food."

"What about popcorn or an oatmeal raisin cookie?" Emma asks.

"Either of those would be a better choice. How about one of each?" asks Mom

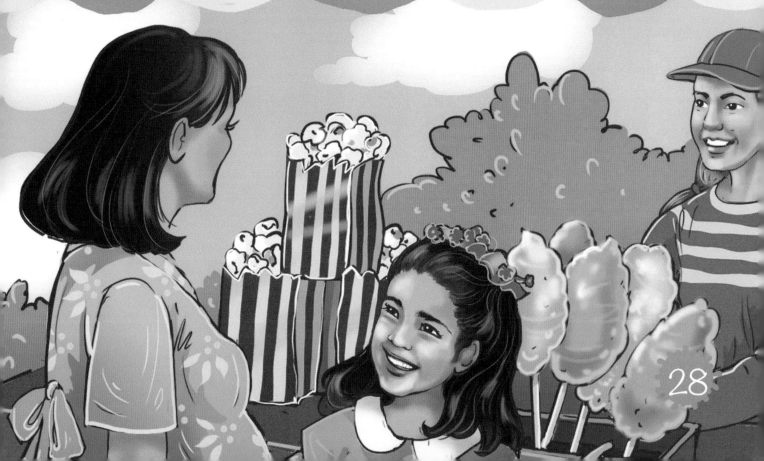

28

"Wow," says another parent in line. "How do you get your kids to make such healthy food choices? Mine always go for the sweets."

"Well," says Emma's mom, "teaching her about the effects of good and bad food on the bacteria inside her makes a big difference."

"I heard you mention something about bugs. Is that what you're referring to?"

"Yes," replies Emma's mom. "When I say "bugs" I'm referring to the bacteria and other microbes that live in us, mostly in our colon. It's referred to as the MICROBIOME. Certain types of food help diversify different good species while other foods promote the kind that can harm us. For optimal health and performance, we need to feed the good bugs what they need which includes many different types of FIBER. The more diverse the fiber we eat, the better it is for us."

"That is very interesting," says the other mom.

"Give me your phone number and I will text you links to start learning about the MICROBIOME and how important it is to take care of our bugs," says Emma's mom.

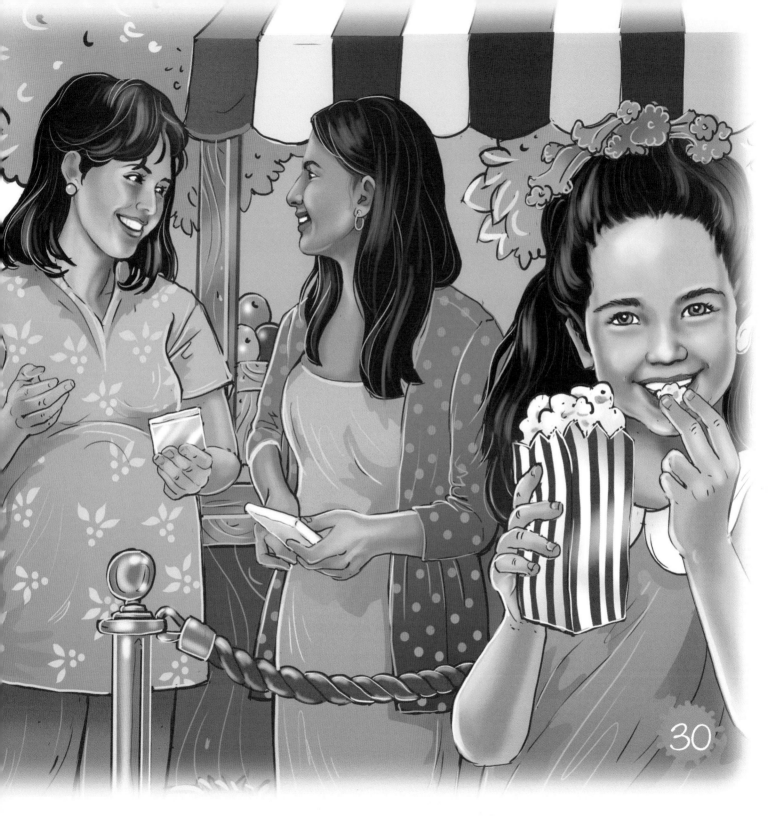

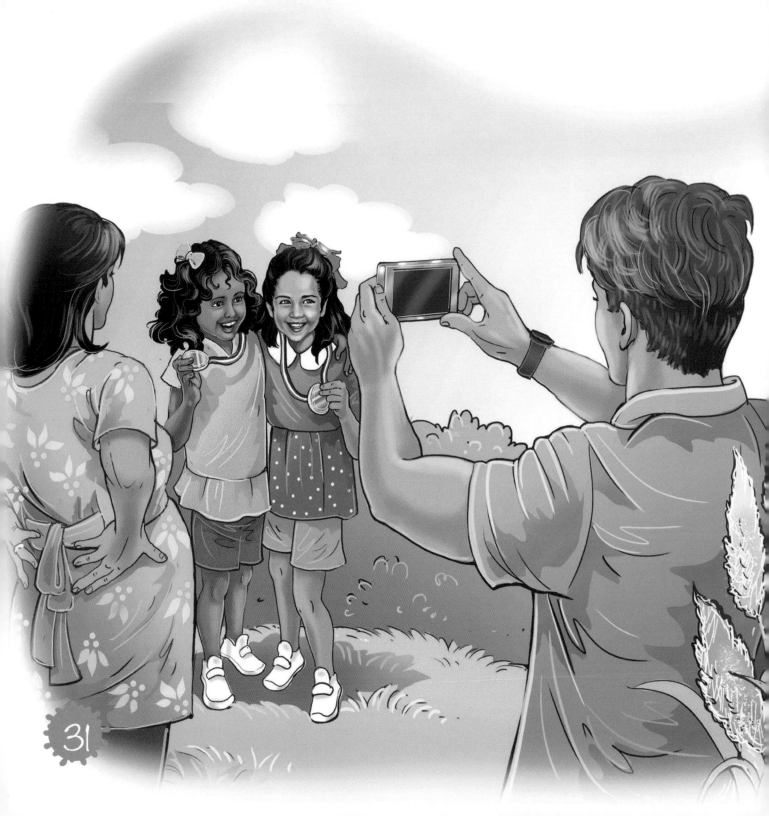

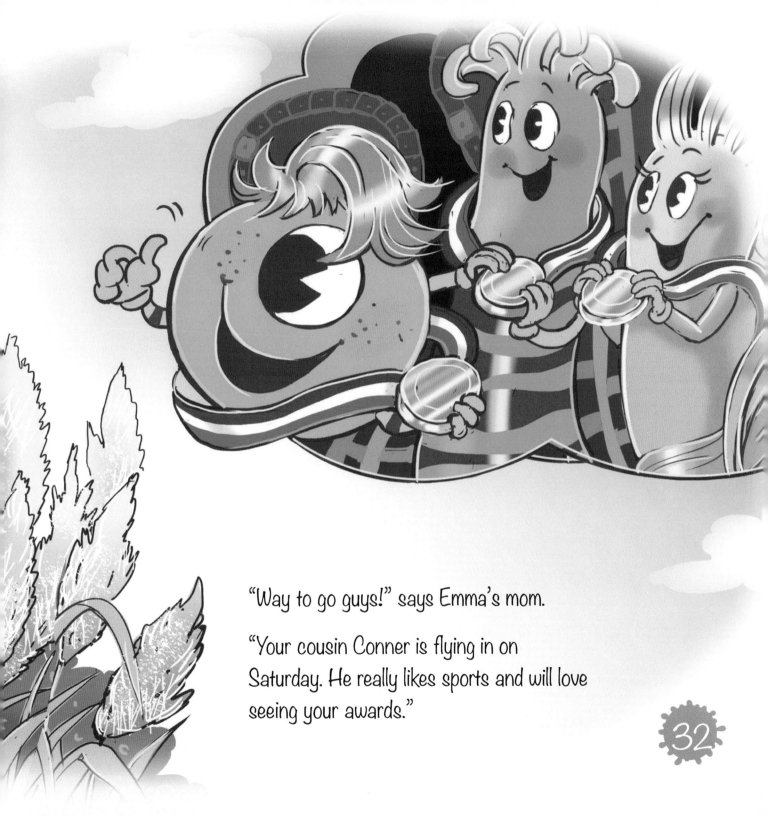

"Way to go guys!" says Emma's mom.

"Your cousin Conner is flying in on Saturday. He really likes sports and will love seeing your awards."

32

"Hi Conner!" says Emma's dad. "It's so good to see you! Have you been training for football? What is the name of your new high school team again?"

"We are the Eagles," says Conner. "Yes. I've been getting ready by running and doing push-ups."

"That's great!" says Emma's mom. "It looks like you have grown a few inches. How tall are you now?"

"I don't know, but Mom says I'm eating them out of house and home!"

Emma laughs. "I hope you're eating food that your belly bugs like if you want to be a good football player."

"Belly bugs? What's she talking about?"

"We've been teaching Emma about the MICROBIOME" her dad explains.

"What's a MICROBIOME?" Conner asks.

"Well, micro means small and biome means life.

Put them together and you get small life."

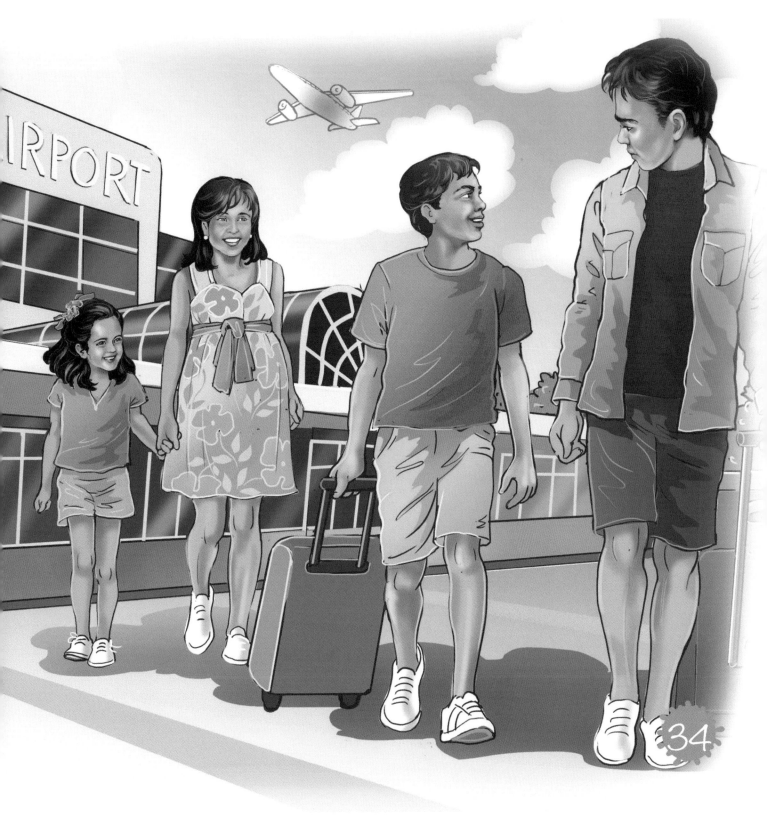
34

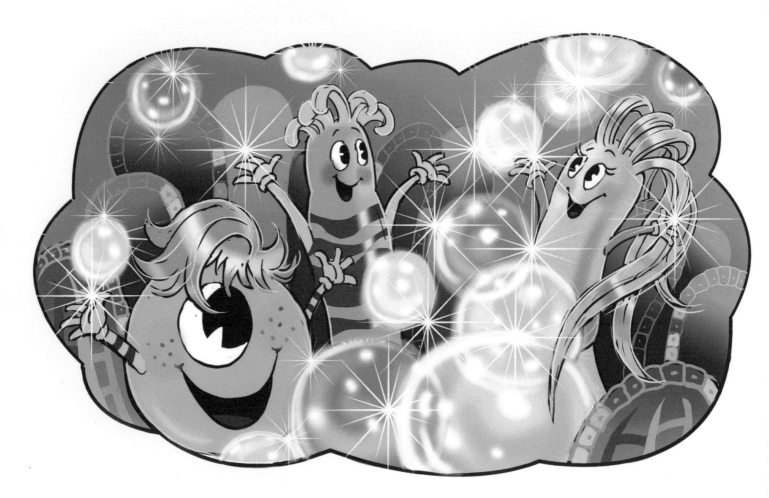

"What kind of life?" Conner asks.

"The kind made up of different species of bacteria. They live all over our body, but most of them are in our intestines and colon. The good bacteria thrive when we eat certain kinds of food that are high in **FIBER**. They produce many great things like **SMALL CHAIN FATTY ACIDS**."

35

"Scientists are just learning how much they help us. We know they keep our **GUT BARRIER** strong to keep toxins out of our blood. They also produce the chemicals for our brain that keep our thoughts happy and healthy. It's a very exciting time in science and medicine. Every day they are learning more about the benefit of a healthy MICROBIOME."

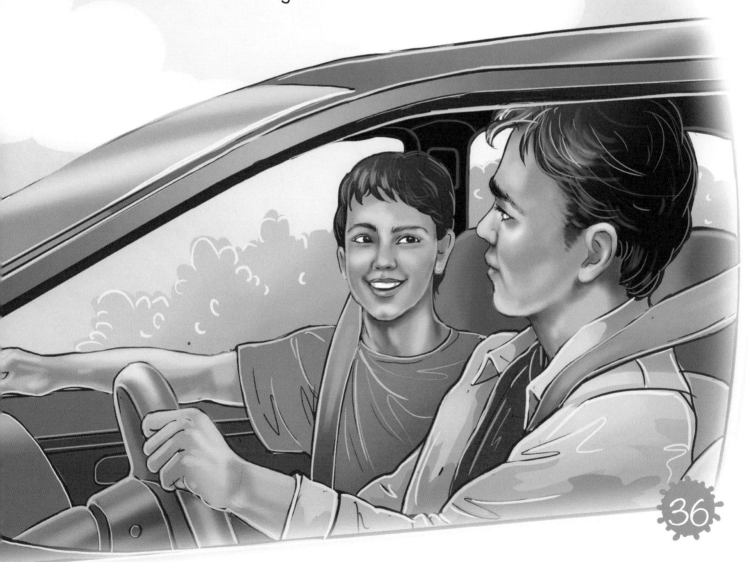

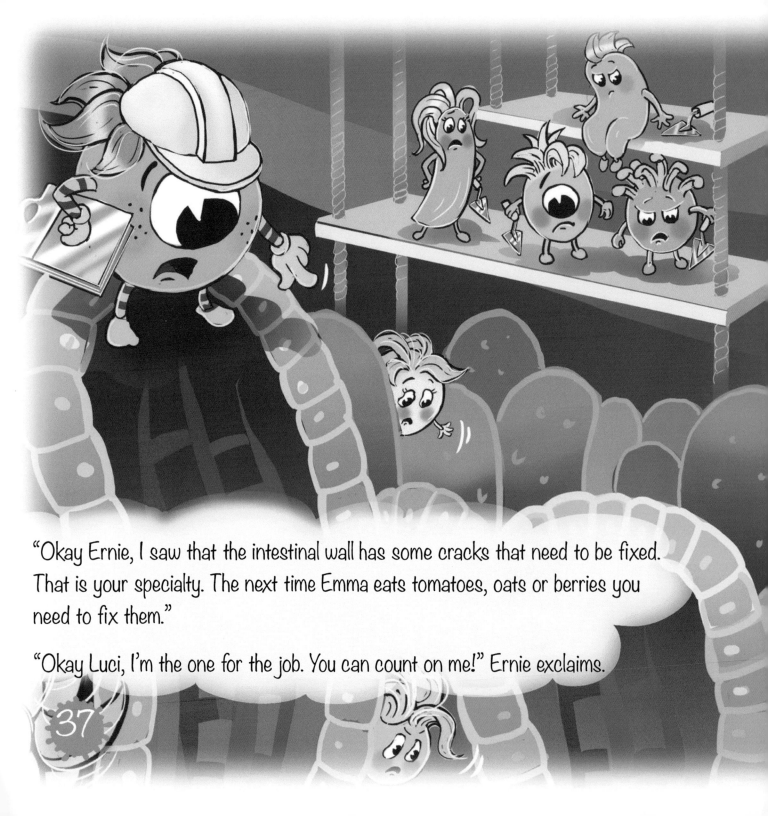

"Okay Ernie, I saw that the intestinal wall has some cracks that need to be fixed. That is your specialty. The next time Emma eats tomatoes, oats or berries you need to fix them."

"Okay Luci, I'm the one for the job. You can count on me!" Ernie exclaims.

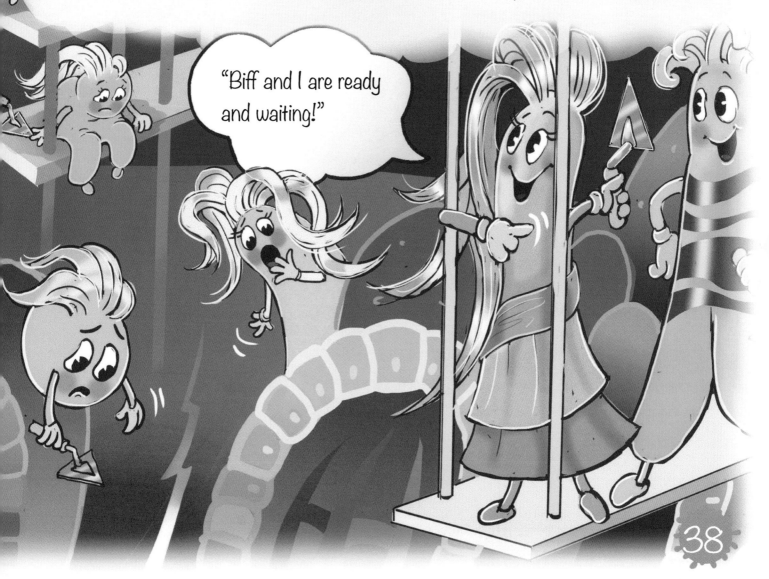

"What will happen if she doesn't eat the right food?" another bacterium asks.
"Well, the lining could break down and ENDOTOXINS could get into Emma's bloodstream." "What are ENDOTOXINS?"
"They're chemicals that can hurt her immune system and keep her from doing her best."

"Biff and I are ready and waiting!"

38

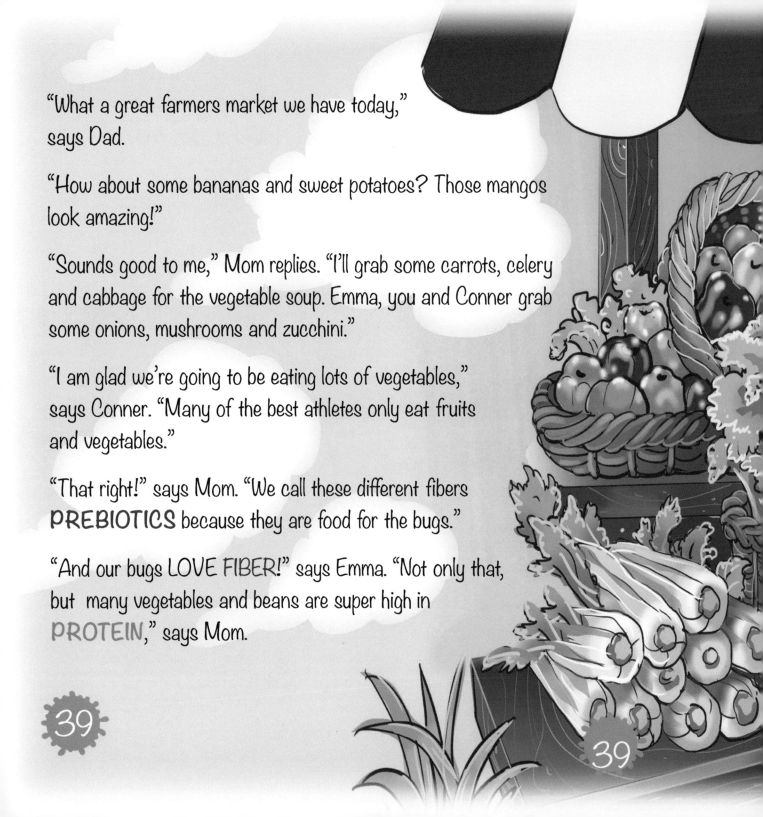

"What a great farmers market we have today," says Dad.

"How about some bananas and sweet potatoes? Those mangos look amazing!"

"Sounds good to me," Mom replies. "I'll grab some carrots, celery and cabbage for the vegetable soup. Emma, you and Conner grab some onions, mushrooms and zucchini."

"I am glad we're going to be eating lots of vegetables," says Conner. "Many of the best athletes only eat fruits and vegetables."

"That right!" says Mom. "We call these different fibers **PREBIOTICS** because they are food for the bugs."

"And our bugs LOVE FIBER!" says Emma. "Not only that, but many vegetables and beans are super high in PROTEIN," says Mom.

39

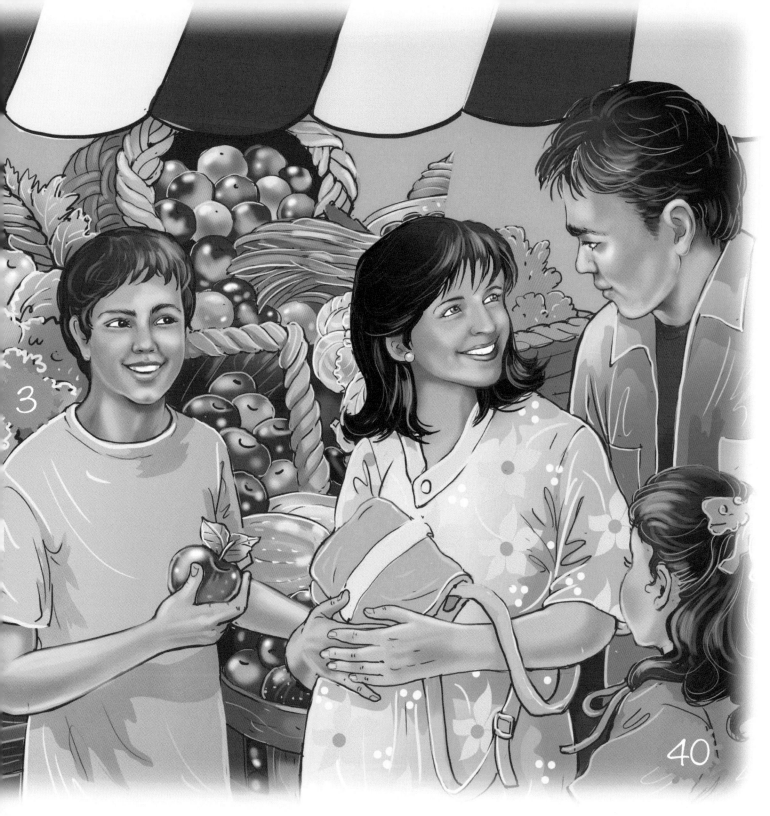

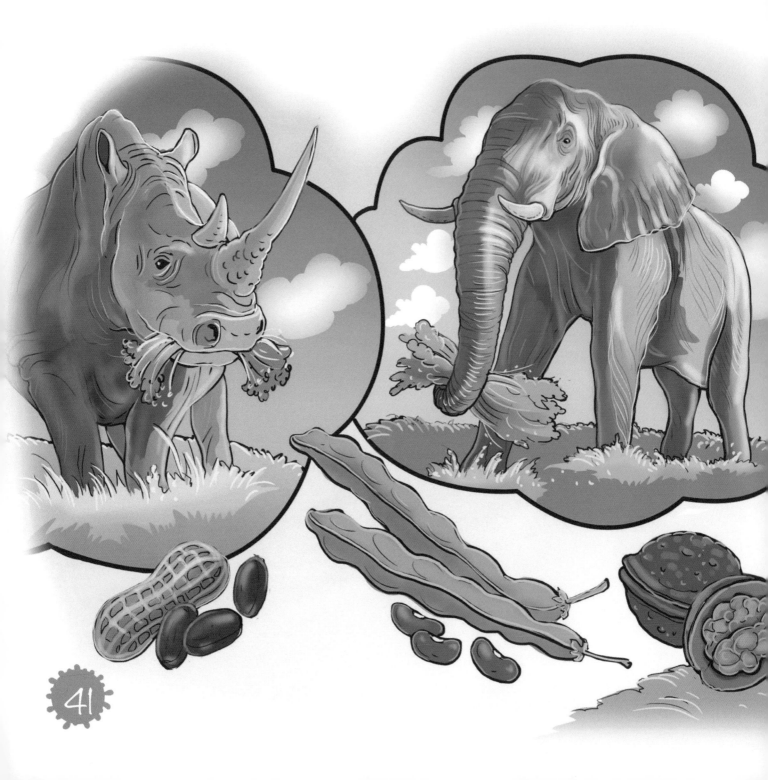

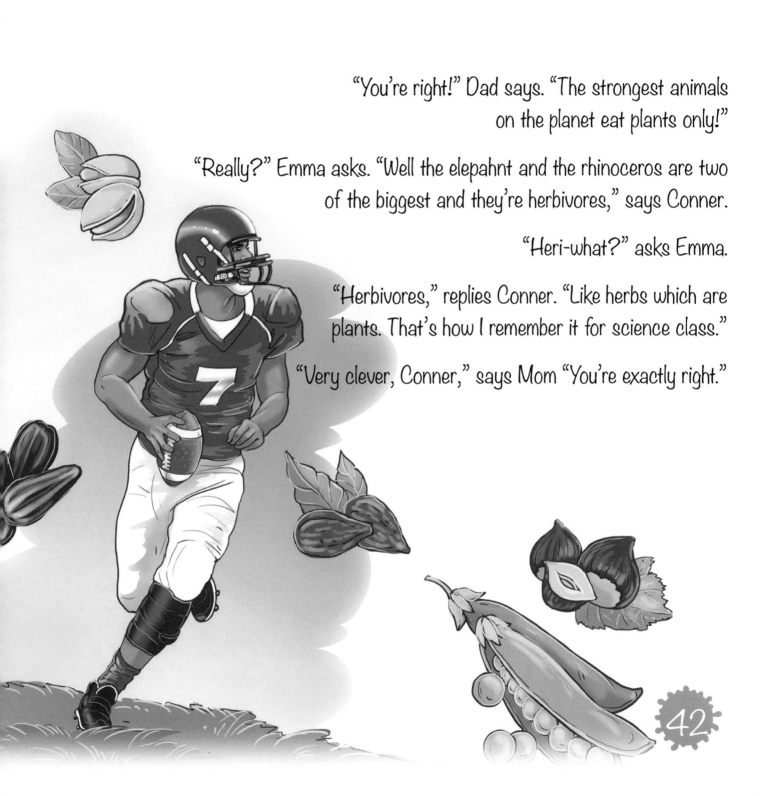

"You're right!" Dad says. "The strongest animals on the planet eat plants only!"

"Really?" Emma asks. "Well the elepahnt and the rhinoceros are two of the biggest and they're herbivores," says Conner.

"Heri-what?" asks Emma.

"Herbivores," replies Conner. "Like herbs which are plants. That's how I remember it for science class."

"Very clever, Conner," says Mom "You're exactly right."

42

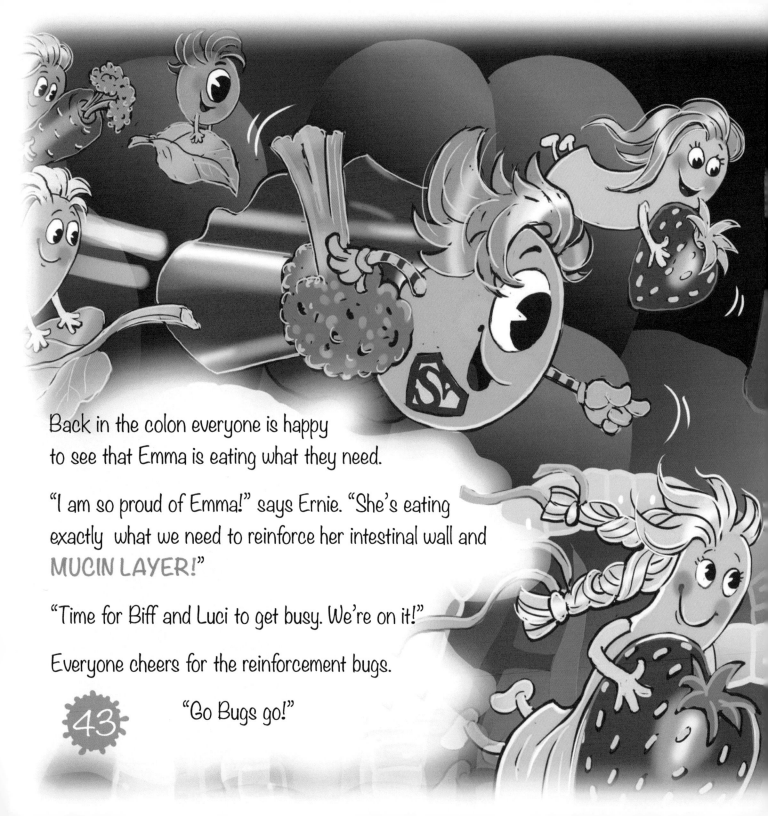

Back in the colon everyone is happy
to see that Emma is eating what they need.

"I am so proud of Emma!" says Ernie. "She's eating
exactly what we need to reinforce her intestinal wall and
MUCIN LAYER!"

"Time for Biff and Luci to get busy. We're on it!"

Everyone cheers for the reinforcement bugs.

43   "Go Bugs go!"

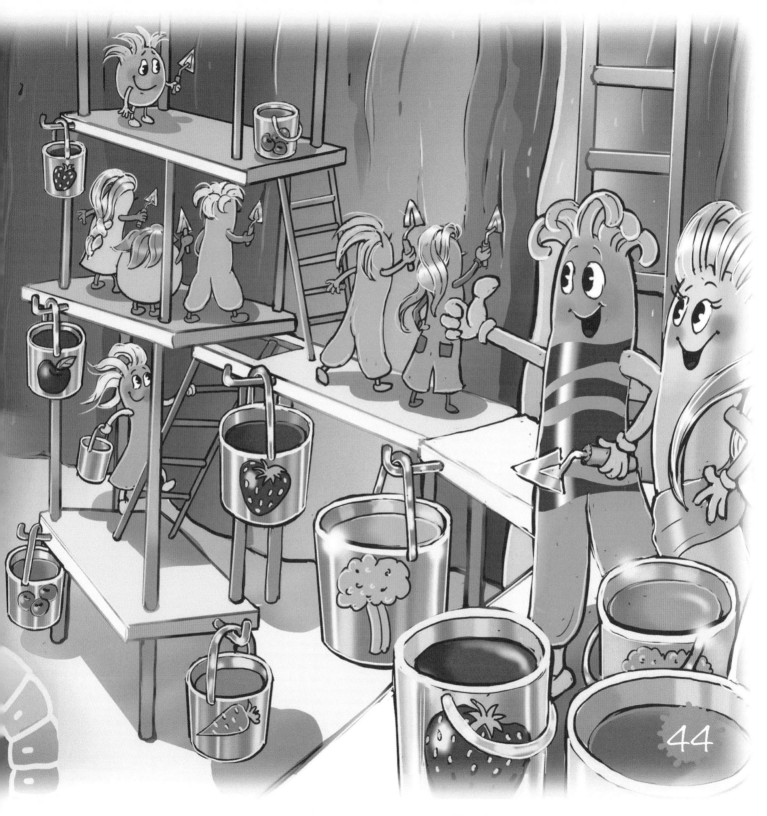

44

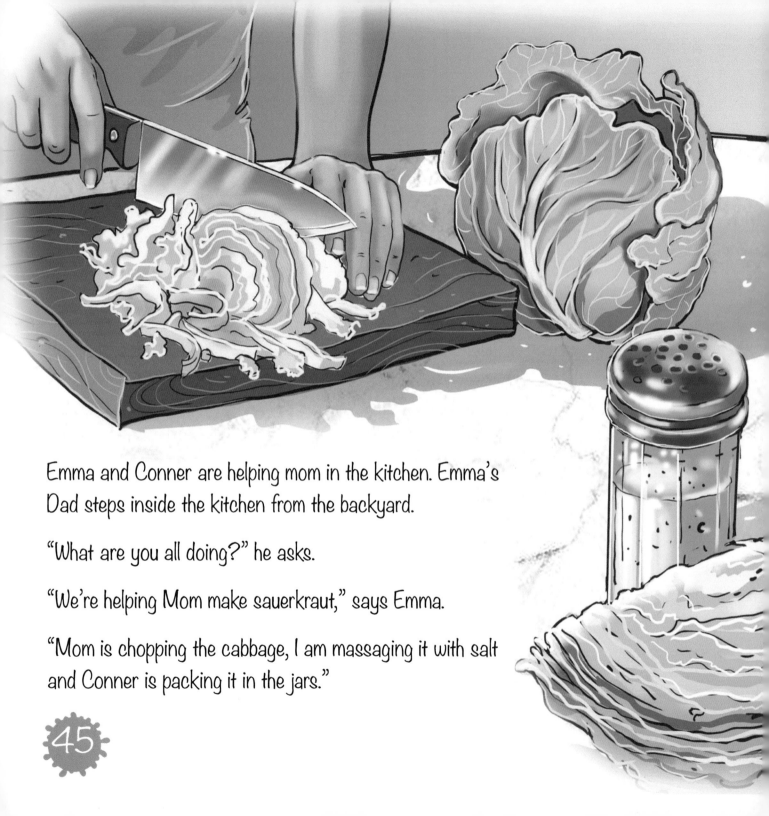

Emma and Conner are helping mom in the kitchen. Emma's Dad steps inside the kitchen from the backyard.

"What are you all doing?" he asks.

"We're helping Mom make sauerkraut," says Emma.

"Mom is chopping the cabbage, I am massaging it with salt and Conner is packing it in the jars."

45

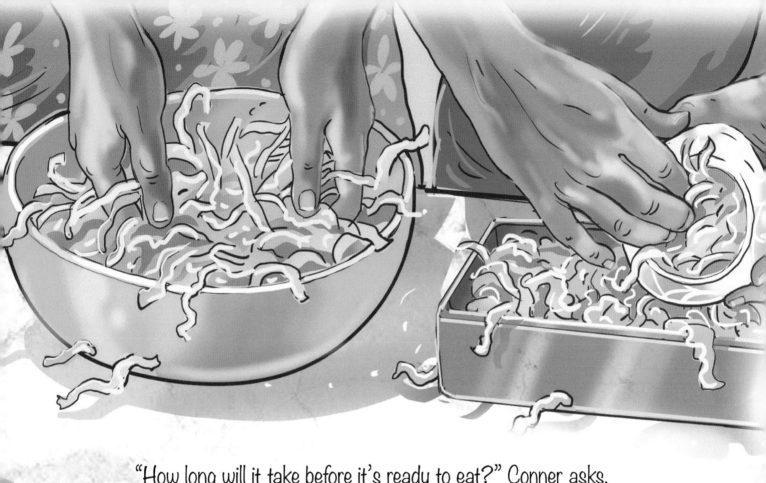

"How long will it take before it's ready to eat?" Conner asks.

"It has to ferment for about two weeks," says Mom.

"Belly bugs LOVE foods like sauerkraut and kombucha because they add different kinds of bacteria to the community. We call them PROBIOTICS."

"When you're all finished helping Mom can you help me out in the garden?" asks Dad.

"Sure," says Conner.

Emma, her dad and Conner are working in the garden.

"What do you need us to do?" Conner asks.

"We need to do some weeding, so the weeds don't take over the garden and keep the plants from growing," Dad explains.

"Current science shows that it's the same way in our gut. Weeds are like the bad bugs that try to take over the good ones that protect us.

That's why we focus on eating healthy food which strengthens

the good bugs and keeps the bad bugs from taking over."

47

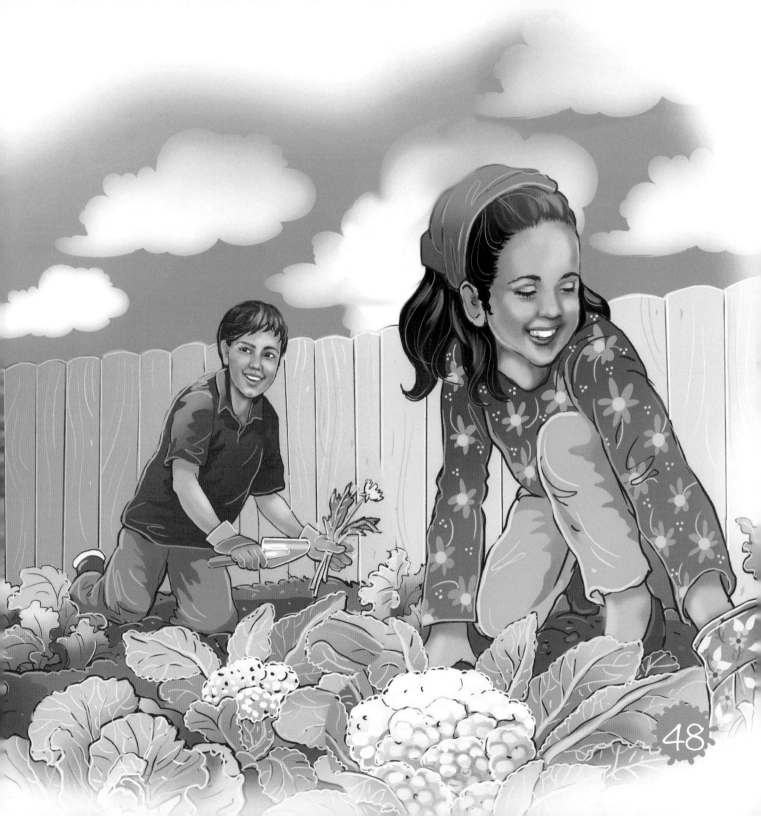

48

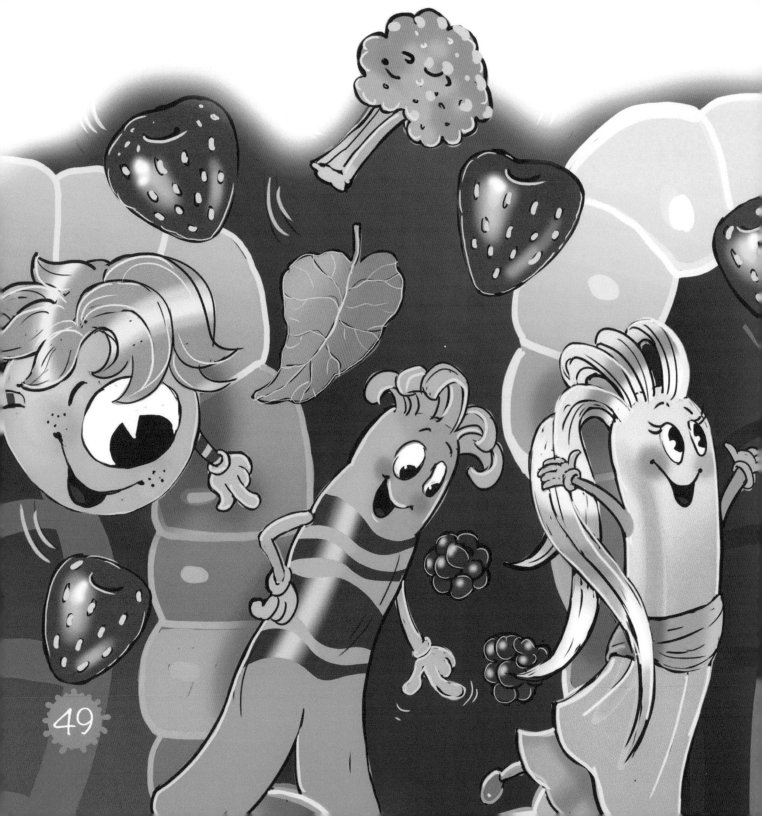

49

"Well, everyone," says Biff. "I am really proud of you all working together to keep Emma's cell wall secure. If she keeps making good healthy choices, we'll be able to do our best work."

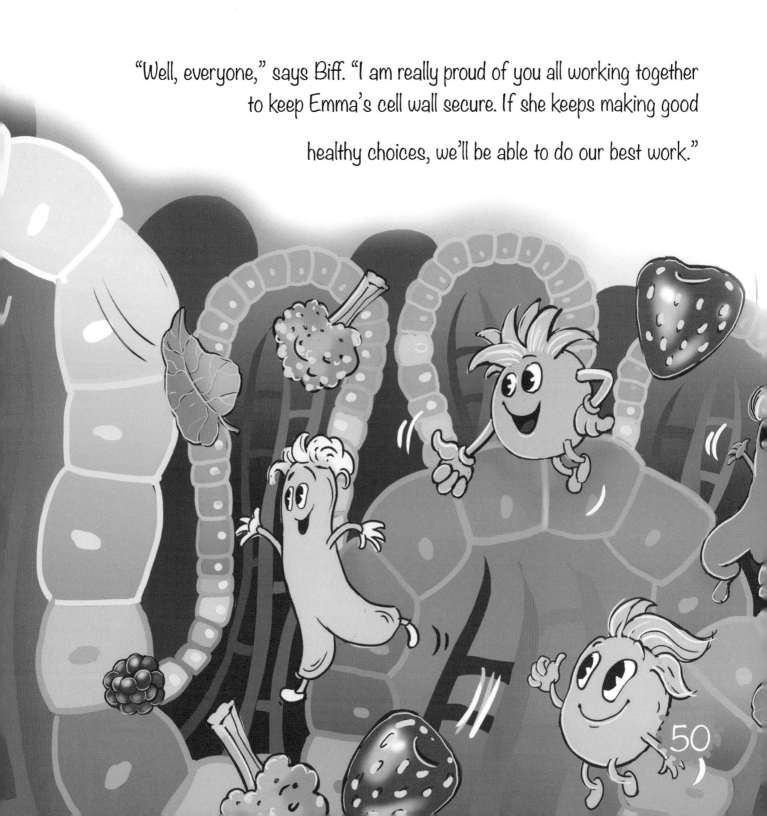

50

"Conner, it's been great having you stay with us this week. We're really going to miss you," says Mom.

"Thanks for teaching me more about my bugs," says Conner.

"I'll focus on keeping them happy when deciding what to eat. Now I understand why some top athletes only eat fruits and vegetables."

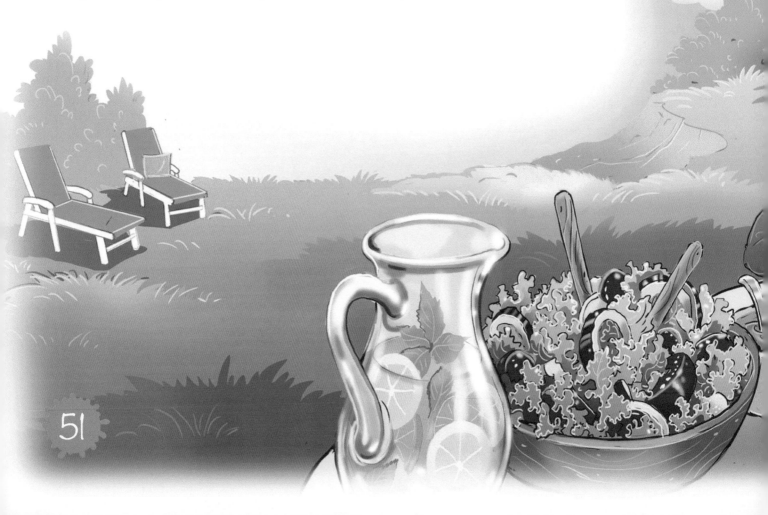

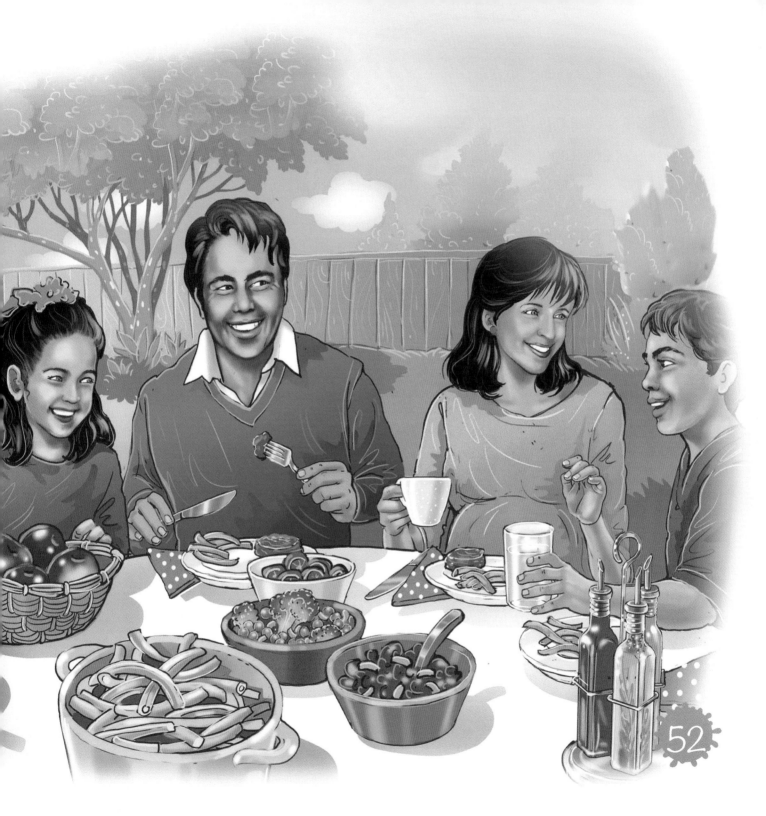
52

Meanwhile, in Conner's colon:

"Wow! I am so happy Conner spent the week at Emma's house. Now we are REALLY happy bugs because of what he's been feeding us," says "Arthur" (Akkermansia).

"If he keeps this up, we'll be able to help him be the best football player on the team. Go eagles!" shouts "Buddy" (Bacillus).

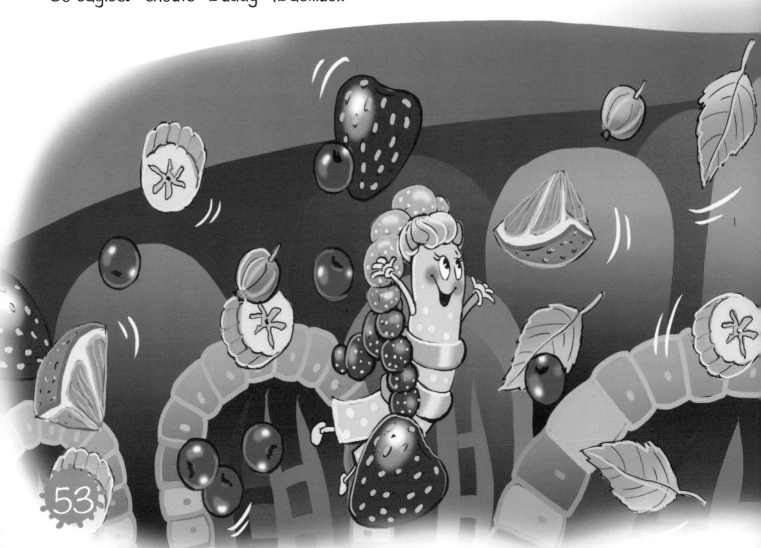

53

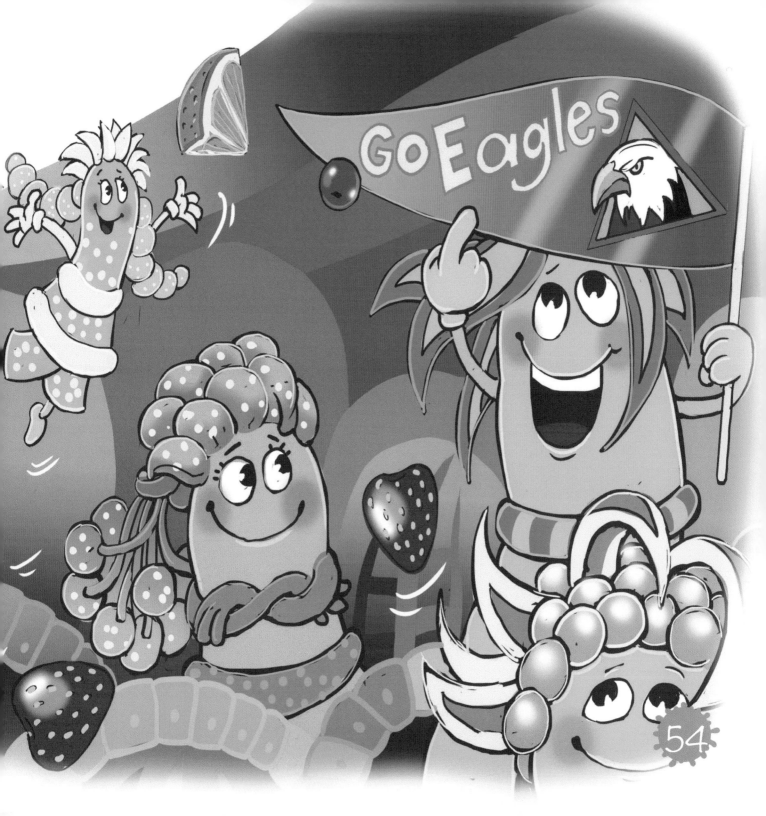

Printed in Great Britain
by Amazon